7 SECRETS YOU NEED TO KNOW ABOUT CANCER

A step-by-step guide to beat cancer

Navodipa B

ISBN: 978-93-5980-003-5

DEDICATION

This book is dedicated to my father-in-law, Mr.
Mahendra Kumar Bagchi

CONTENTS

PREFACE

There is a relentless call for awareness in the shadows of uncertainty and fear where cancer profoundly impacts lives. The book is a beacon of hope, shedding light on cancer's many challenges and triumphs and how the human spirit can overcome adversity. Sharing stories of courage, resilience, and scientific breakthroughs, we explore how this disease works. Combining knowledge, compassion, and a collective commitment, we aim to empower ourselves and others to fight cancer together. It is an invitation to build awareness, support, and hope together.

PROLOGUE

Having just returned from their honeymoon, Ayaan and Naina eagerly embraced their new life together. Destiny, however, had other plans. Their world was shattered by a late-night phone call just before they resumed their normal routine. Unforeseen and daunting, the news was a wake-up call they never expected. Despite uncertainty and fear, they stood together, determined to unravel the mystery. It is an inspiring journey through cancer awareness, where the strength of togetherness is tested. This book is a tale of love, resilience, and the pursuit of answers.

INTRODUCTION: UNDERSTANDING CANCER

It was a Sunday night. Ayaan was planning to go to sleep when his phone rang. "Maa," the phone screen popped up. It was quite late, and his mom knew he had to return to the office the next day. He is returning after the long leave he took for his marriage. 'Answer it,' said Naina, his newly-wed wife beside him.

'Hello! What happened, Maa?'

Ayaan's face turned pale while listening to the other side of the phone. "Dad is in the hospital," he told Naina. He was overwhelmed by the news and didn't know what to do. They have just come back a few days back. Naina looked for flight tickets and booked whichever flight was available. Ayaan left for home at 1:15 AM, and that's how it all started.

* * *

1. Cancer- the villain

What comes to your mind when you hear someone suffering from cancer? Maybe you start feeling sad about the patient; maybe you imagine how much pain they are going through. But most of all, you feel 'fear.' A fear of losing that person. Why do people have this fear of cancer? Because we fear what we don't know about. We believe there is no cure for cancer, hence the fear. Let's start knowing about cancer to understand the problem and dismiss the fear.

1.1. Cancer-the disease

Our body is made up of trillions of cells. Many of these cells die each day because of their age, and new cells are generated and replaced at their places. This process happens because our body needs these cells to function properly. Now imagine if some of these cells stopped dying and became immortal because of some abnormality caused in our system; what would be the consequences? The number of cells would increase, leading to abnormal growth in the body, causing a tumor. The extra growth is stopped if the body understands and rectifies the problem. What if our body fails to do so? After a certain time, these unwanted growth or tumor cells will not be able to fit inside one small tissue, and the tumor will burst, releasing the abnormal cells into our system. These cells can travel to any body part, creating a new tumor and repeating the same process. This condition is called cancer.

1.2. Why does cancer happen

The new cells are generated in our body by cell division. Some specific factors or genes control the generation of new cells and the dying of old cells. If there is any abnormality in those genes, cancer can happen. The abnormality can happen by some error during our lifetime or some error that came to us genetically. The abnormality that we are talking about is some change in the genes. This process of introducing any change in our genes is called mutation. This change can occur anytime and anywhere in the body. Sometimes our system recognizes the change and repairs it.

Sometimes it fails to do so, leading to uncontrolled cell division or immortality of the cells, causing cancer.

1.3. Carcinogens

Who will be at higher risk of facing a road accident? One who goes out every day or who does not go out often. Of course, the chances are much higher for the one exposed to the road daily.

Similarly, exposure to certain substances causes a higher risk of changing the genes leading to mutation. These substances are called carcinogens. Cigarettes are one such carcinogen. Some other examples of carcinogens are UV rays from sunlight, automobile exhaust fumes, etc.

1.4. How does cancer develop

There are three ways to develop cancers; first, if the abnormality happens during cell division and is not repaired; second, if the change in the gene is caused by repetitive exposure to carcinogens. And third, if the cancer is inherited in the genes from parents. When cancer develops, the number of cells increases, forming a tumor. These tumors or tissue lumps are called 'benign' tumors. They are harmless and can not be considered cancerous, as they can't spread yet. However, if they start to grow day by day, the organ loses the power to hold these extra masses of tissue. Some cells from the tumor then go on an expedition to find a new place to colonize further. Then the tumor becomes cancerous, and that is how it spreads. These tumors, which can now spread, are promoted to be called malignant tumors. This condition of tumors moving from one organ to another is called metastasis.

1.5. Stages of cancer

Cancer stages are very popular, and many of us have at least heard about the term. The stages are used to describe cancer and its growth and its spreading in nearby areas. The staging of cancer is done by a system called the TNM system. T=Tumor, N=Lymph Node, and M=Metastasis. Let's talk about them one by one.

T or tumor states the size of the primary tumor, where it is located, and if it is invaded into other organs in the same area. The letter T is often followed by a number that describes the tumor further. For example, TX =No information about the tumor; T0 = No evidence of a tumor; Tis= tumor is only present in the primary tissue and has not spread anywhere else. T1-T4 means the size of the tumor on a scale of 1 to 4. The more the number means, the tumor size and has spread to other body parts.

N or Lymph Nodes are small bean-shaped organs that are present in the different areas of the body. They help in fighting against any germs that enter the body. These lymph nodes are connected throughout our body, like blood circulation. Cancer cells travel through these lymphatic systems, so checking cancer cells at the lymph nodes is important. Cancer cells in lymph nodes indicate if the cancer cells have spread to other body parts.

M or metastasis is when the primary tumor cells have spread to other body parts. So, if the cancer has not spread anywhere, the stage will be M0; if it has spread to other organs, it will be M1.

1.6. Types of cancer

The cancers are named after the organ it has originated from. For example, if cancer grows in the kidney, the person will get kidney cancer. If that cancer spreads to the lungs, it will still be called kidney cancer with secondary lung development. It would not become lung cancer. There are so many types of cells present in our body. Cancer can start anywhere among all these cell types. Broadly, it is categorized into four main types. These are discussed below.

1.6.1. Solid cancers

➢ **Carcinoma**

Carcinoma is when cancer develops in the outer lining cells of any organ in the body. These cells are known as epithelial cells. Some examples of epithelial cells would be skin cells. 80-90% of all cancers are carcinoma. Carcinoma also develops where secretory cells are present such as the breast. Carcinoma is also of the following types:

Ø *Melanoma*

It is a rare type of skin cancer where melanocytes or pigmented cells become cancerous. These can easily be seen in the early stages and are often cured. So, if you find any unwanted "ugly duckling" in your skin growing daily, you might want to see a doctor for a check-up.

Ø *Basal cell carcinoma*

Basal cells are the outermost layer of our skin where new skin cells generate. If there is cancer in this layer, it is called basal cell carcinoma. These tumors look like translucent skin-colored bumps.

Ø *Squamous cell skin cancer*

Squamous cell carcinoma is a cancer formed in the middle and inner layers of the skin. They are usually not life-threatening. But they can be aggressive and cause problems if they remain untreated.

Ø *Merkel cell carcinoma*

This condition is a cancer developed beneath the skin or in a hair follicle. The tumor looks like small, smooth, shiny lumps on the skin. The tumor is often colored pink, red, or blue. They are highly prone to spreading in other parts of the body.

- **Sarcoma**

Sarcoma is when cancer develops in the connective tissues of the body. Connective tissues are the tissues that connect different organs. They provide support and protection to the body. They also help in the movement of nutrients. Mainly these tissues store fat. Some examples of connective tissues would be bones and cartilage. Sarcoma also is of different types, which are as follows.

Ø *Soft tissue sarcoma*

Soft tissues are the tissues that hold our body together. They include muscles, tendons, blood vessels, nerves, etc. A cancer in any of them is called soft tissue sarcoma. Early stages of soft tissue sarcoma are very difficult to diagnose. They are commonly developed into arms and legs. Specific organs such as the lungs and colon are also soft but not soft tissues.

Ø *Osteosarcoma*

Osteosarcoma is a cancer in the bones. Mostly this cancer happens in young adults or teenagers. Sometimes children also get the disease. The symptoms include swelling near a bone or breaking of a bone for no reason. Very rarely, osteosarcoma can happen in soft tissues as well.

Ø *Ewing's sarcoma*

This cancer is also a type of bone cancer where cancer develops from a specialized type of bone cells. It is often observed in young adults. This type of cancer results in pain near the tumor area.

Ø *Chondrosarcoma*

Chondrosarcoma is a cancer in the cartilage. Cartilage is the tough and flexible structure that makes up many structures in the body, such as the nose and ear. They are also present at the joints of the bones, providing a cushion effect. Pain and swelling are the common symptoms of this cancer.

1.6.2. Liquid cancers

- **Lymphoma**

Lymphoma is a cancer developed in any part of the lymphatic system. The lymphatic system is our body's sewage system, which cleans our system. It maintains the body fluid by moving a colorless fluid called lymph. This system is responsible for our body's immunity and production of white blood cells. Lymphoma is of the following types:

Ø *Hodgkin's lymphoma*

This type of lymphoma originated from a special type of white blood cell called the lymphocytes. They are specialized cancer cells with some specific characteristics, including the presence of more than one nucleus. Hodgkin's lymphoma is an aggressive cancer that can spread faster. However, the treatment for Hodgkin's lymphoma is possible.

Ø *Non-Hodgkin's lymphoma*

Non-Hodgkin's lymphoma is any type of cancer originating in the lymphatic system other than Hogdkin's. They also originate from specialized white blood cells. As it is also a group of many cancers formed in the lymph, the aggressiveness varies among different types and stages.

Ø *Cutaneous lymphoma*

Cutaneous lymphoma is rare in which a specific white blood cell called a T-lymphocyte cell becomes cancerous. These cells are very important fighters of our immune system. In healthy conditions, whenever some foreign entity attacks our body, our immune system generates a troop of these T-lymphocyte cells that fight that particular intruder. However, they are directed against our skin cells in case of this cancer condition.

- **Leukemia**

Leukemia is also known as blood cancer grown in the bone marrow. Bone marrow is the soft spongy tissue found at the central part of the bones that produces red blood cells, white blood cells, and platelets. Red blood cells are important for the oxygen supply in our body. White blood cells are responsible for the body's defense. The platelets help in blood clotting to prevent bleeding. Cancer in the bone marrow produces cancerous immortal blood cells. There are several types of leukemia. They are as follows:

Ø *Acute lymphocytic leukemia*

This type of blood cancer grows during the maturation of early white blood cells, the lymphocytes. This cancer starts in bone marrow or blood, and then it spreads. The term acute means it is highly aggressive and can spread within one or two months.

Ø *Acute myeloid leukemia*

This type of blood cancer results in the formation of abnormal and immature white blood cells. They are called myoblast cells. As these cells are numerous in the body, there is less room for healthy blood cells. So, the patient becomes prone to other infections due to a lack of healthy and mature white blood cells.

Ø *Agnogenic myeloid leukemia*

In this type of specialized cancer, the bone marrow gets replaced by some other tissue. So, the blood can not be formed in the bone marrow. Hence blood is formed by organs like the spleen and liver. As a result, these organs become overloaded with the extra work of producing so much blood for the body's normal functioning. Also, it is not possible to remain healthy with such abnormality.

Ø *Chronic lymphocytic leukemia*

In this cancer, only the lymphocyte numbers increase rapidly. The detection of this cancer is very tricky at an early stage.

Ø *Chronic myeloid leukemia*

White blood cells are mainly of two types; one with many granules and another without. The ones with the granules are called granulocytes. In chronic myeloid leukemia, these granulocytes increase in number.

Ø *Essential thrombocythemia*

In this type of leukemia, the number of platelets becomes uncontrollably high. Platelets help in clot formation when there is a wound in the body in healthy conditions. But in this case, the chances of forming a blood clot within the blood vessels are pretty high. That clot can travel through the blood vessels. The person can get a heart attack if it goes to the heart. If it travels to the brain, a brain stroke can happen. So this cancer harms the body and increases the risk of heart attack, stroke, etc.

Ø *Myelodysplastic syndromes*

In this type of blood cancer, the blood cells do not mature. They are generated and remain immature, so they become useless. Patients with this type of leukemia always feel tired, get infected easily, and become very weak.

• **Myeloma**

Myeloma is a special type of cancer where the cancer is developed in the plasma cells of bone marrow. Plasma cells are a type of white blood cells present in the bone marrow. When healthy, these plasma cells aggressively eat up foreign particles entering our body. Myeloma is also of two types:

Ø *Plasmacytoma*

This type of cancer develops in plasma cells in one bone.

Ø *Multiple myeloma*

In multiple myeloma, cancer is present in multiple bones.

1.7. How quickly does cancer grow

Cancer is an umbrella of several types of diseases. By now, we have an idea that there are 2 types of cancer. First is solid cancer, with a solid mass or tumor present. In contrast, the second type is liquid cancer, such as blood, lymph, and myeloma or bone marrow plasma cell cancer. So, the spreading speed of all types of cancers will also vary. There are some cancers where a tumor grows slowly and takes years to spread. At the same time, some cancers are very aggressive as well.

You can imagine the cancer cells as someone who has to leave his home country and travel to another country to settle down without a visa. If anything goes wrong, he will not be able to achieve his goal. Similarly, cancer cells must undergo certain steps to spread and settle down to a different body part. These steps are:

- The cancer cell must change to grow and invade the normal tissue.
- Next, they must bypass the human immune system like the police.
- Then they have to travel to the nearest lymph node for further spreading. Lymph acts like their road to travel.
- They have to anchor some new place to settle in.
- Finally, they have to grow a new tumor at that new place.

All the cancer cells that are spreading must undergo all these steps. It takes work. So, the speed or aggressiveness of cancer depends on the type of cancer, the stage of cancer, and, last but not least, the individual patient's immune system.

1.8. Can cancer be infected

Cancer is a disease where cells grow uncontrollably because of the abnormality in the genes.

It's not the common cold you can 'catch' from someone with cancer. But cancer can be infected by a virus called human papillomavirus. This virus is a sexually transmitted infection that causes cancer in the genital regions in most cases. Vaccine for this virus is available, and teenagers are recommended to get vaccinated. One should be careful before selecting a partner to prevent human papillomavirus infection.

1.9. Is cancer genetic?

Cancer is a condition caused by genetic abnormalities. So, it is pretty clear that cancer is genetic. But there is a catch of cancer being a genetic disease. The exact cancerous tumor cells are not passed down to the child from the parents.

Suppose a normal cell wants to become cancerous one day. In that case, it has to undergo a 'training program' or a series of 'changes' or 'mutations' to become a cancer cell. A normal cell to become cancerous takes at least seven mutations or genetic changes. In most cases, the cells already have three to four mutations inherited from the parents, increasing cancer risk. But it does not mean everyone in a family will get a specific type of cancer.

1.10. Who is prone to cancer

As discussed in the previous section, a cell must undergo several changes before becoming cancerous. A person exposed to more carcinogens is more likely to develop cancer. There are other factors as well that increase the risk of developing cancer. They are age, lifestyle, food, family history, habits, and environment. Each of them is discussed in detail in the later chapters.

*   *   *

SECRET NO. 1: DETECT CANCER EARLY

"How are you feeling now?"- asked the doctor while examining Mr. Rao. Ayaan was beside his hospital bed. "He has been vomiting since last night. Why is this happening" he asked the doctor. 'We are doing some blood tests. Will be able to tell something once the results come,' said the doctor and left. The next day blood test results came, and reports were normal. Ayaan discharged Mr. Rao, and they came home, relieved, until nine months later when his health deteriorated again.

"I'm afraid your father has cancer, Mr. Ayaan," said the doctor. Ayaan became numb when he heard the term 'cancer'. The doctor must have confused my father with another patient. "But he is here because of jaundice and not cancer!" he said to the doctor. How can he have cancer all of a sudden? He thought. Besides, how can his father get cancer? He never smoked or drank alcohol. The doctor replied that the jaundice was happening because of the cancer. He can't believe his ears. Why him, of all people? After a long pause, he asked the doctor what needed to be done.

* * *

2. Police vs. thief - cancer detection

Our body's immune system is like a group of highly qualified police officers who patrol each part of the body. They are always alert about any unknown or foreign material entering our system. They always follow the law and do whatever they can to protect the innocent cells of our bodies. But cancer cells are like some mischievous gangsters who pretend to be innocent in front of these police officers. Cancer cells are not foreign to our body, so our immune system often does not recognize them as a threat.

2.1. Why is it so difficult to detect cancer early?

Whenever our immune system feels something is wrong or some foreign particle has entered our body, it sends signals. For example, when some allergic response happens to us, we develop symptoms like redness, swelling, etc. These are known as inflammatory responses. Why does this happen? It is because our immune system alerts our system that something is wrong. But cancer is a part of our body. So, distinguishing them from normal innocent cells is difficult.

2.2. Early symptoms of cancer

When cancer develops in any part of our body, we normally feel nothing. Spotting cancer at an early stage is a tough job. Our 24/7, tireless immune system also can not spot cancer even after working and living with the cancer cells. But just because it is a tough job does not mean we will not even try to spot cancer at an early stage. After all, our ignorance can become life-threatening for us. Let's discuss some common symptoms that cancer patients develop before getting diagnosed.

- Early symptoms of any cancer can be some persistent changes in the body. For example, feeling fatigued. Cancer takes up much energy to nourish ourselves, so most patients feel chronic fatigue. So, any change that feels unusual can be an early cancer symptom. Other persistent changes can include heartburn, urination pattern, a change in bowel movement, any type of bleeding for unknown reasons, and so on.
- Another very common cancer symptom is weight gain or loss for no reason. Most cancer patients lose a lot of weight when they have cancer.
- The formation of any kind of lump which does not feel normal might be an early sign of cancer.
- Any change in any existing mole or growing new moles can also be an early cancer symptom. Sometimes these moles change their color or start bleeding.
- Skin soreness, itchy skin, fever, night sweats, headache, and jaundice can also be early signs of cancer.
- Any pain that persists for days or weeks after can be a cancer symptom.

The discussed symptoms are not always the only symptoms of cancer and can result from something else. But, it is always better not to ignore these symptoms so that the treatment can be started early.

2.3. How to detect cancer early

When cancer develops, the patient often starts to feel weak. The tumor takes up most of the energy one gets to grow these extra cells. The most important factor is awareness to detect cancer early. One has to be well aware of their body. So that if any change happens, one can consult a doctor. Even if some unusual lump in your body is not painful, don't wait for the pain to occur and consult a doctor as soon as possible. The earliest cancer detection is only possible if the patient is always alert about his body and does not ignore even the smallest but persistent changes. The early detection of cancer requires three steps.

Diagnosis

Diagnosis is the first step when someone needs to consult a doctor. The doctor then suggests further tests for specific cancer detection.

Screening

Screening is a procedure for quick scans of specific organs for cancers. For example, mammography is done for breast cancer testing, and a CT scan is done for lung cancer detection. Screening can give an idea of any unusual growth in our body.

Testing for genetic risks

As cancer can run in some families, understanding the risk of getting cancer is also important. In this way, one can be aware of their chances of getting specific cancers and avoid the risk factors accordingly.

2.4. Detection of different cancers

Some very common early signs of specific cancers are listed below.

Skin cancer

Presence of scars or moles that grow with time, itchy skin with sores. Sores that are persistent and not healing for a long time. Any smooth pink bump or a lump with blood vessels inside.

Breast cancer

Presence of any lump near the breasts, a dented nipple, or unusual nipple discharge that is not breast milk. Any unusual mass that pains. Swelling in breasts, pain, irritation, etc.

Lung cancer

Coughing that does not go away, losing weight, frequent headache, blood clots, coughing up blood, bone pain, shortness of breath, not feeling hungry, constant chest pain.

Kidney cancer

Blood in the urine, pain in the lower abdomen for no known reason, lump at one side of the back, tiredness, loss of appetite, fever, anemia, losing weight.

Prostrate cancer

Difficulty in urination starting and holding back, blood in urine, burning sensation during urination, needing to pee often, especially at night, and pain in the lower back, hips, and thighs.

Colon or rectal cancer

Losing weight, feeling weak, persistent change in bowel movement, constipation or diarrhea that last more than a few days, Constant feeling pressure in the rectum, stomach pain, and blood in the stool.

Melanoma

Presence of any mark on the skin with asymmetrical or uneven edges, any mole that is quickly growing or changing shape, a mole larger than the tip of a pencil eraser, any scar or mole that bleeds or itches.

Bladder cancer

Blood in the urine, the urine may look pinkish.

Lymph cancer

Large lymph nodes that might feel like lumps under the skin tired all the time, full after eating small portions of food, chills, fever, night sweats, pain in the chest, and swollen abdomen.

Blood cancer

Fever, chills, night sweats, feeling weak and exhausted all the time, swollen lymph nodes that feels like lumps under the skin, enlarged liver and spleen that might feel like a mass under ribs, tiny red spots on the skin, bone pain, frequent nosebleeds.

Pancreatic cancer

Yellowing of skin or jaundice, feeling exhausted, pain in the upper abdomen or back, developing diabetes.

Liver cancer

Loss of appetite, swollen abdomen, enlarged spleen and liver that feels like a mass under the ribs, vomiting, pain near the right shoulder blade and gut, fainting, constipation, and skin itching for no reason.

Thyroid cancer

Swelling in the front of the neck, trouble swallowing and breathing, voice change, pain in the neck radiating to the ears, constant cough.

Uterine cancer

Abnormal vaginal bleeding, unusual vaginal discharge, pelvic pain, and weight loss.

2.5. Technologies to detect cancer

If some thieves come to your house and steal some valuable stuff, what will be your first step to catch them? You will report them to the police, and they will start investigating. To identify the thieves, you might first examine the place for any evidence they might have left. Then you might want to have their images. For that, you will look for some CCTV footage. Also, you might ask a painting artist to draw images of the thieves depending on the description of some witnesses.

Similarly, when a patient reports the symptoms to a doctor, the doctor would want to look for evidence that cancer might have left. That's why they ask for several tests before declaring what happened. Most of the time, the doctors check some blood test reports. For example, the police are looking for evidence that the thief might have left at the place of the crime as cancer might cause changes in some parameters in our blood. Next, the doctor asks for some image-based tests to see the cancer to check if anything unusual is present. If they find something after a scan of that organ, they check if it is cancerous. The details of these tests are discussed next.

2.6. Blood tests for cancer detection

Blood is the ultimate transport system that cargos things from here to there inside our body. If cancer has to communicate or even wants to go from one tumor to other parts of the body, it must use the blood or the lymph. Even the lymphatic system is well connected to our blood as it cleans the whole body. So, any remains from cancer left in the blood can be useful for us to detect them. This situation is similar to tapping the suspects' telephones to detect who is the thief here. So, the first test a doctor might recommend is a blood test. Not only that, blood tests are affordable and easier for general monitoring of overall physiology. The types of blood tests doctors recommend for cancer detection are discussed below.

Complete/ total blood count

The complete blood count gives us an idea of the total number of red blood cells, white blood cells, and platelets. Certain cancers, like blood and lymph, lead to abnormal numbers of these cell types. Other cancers also can affect the cell count of the blood.

Cancer markers test

Cancer sometimes releases certain substances in the blood, which helps in cancer detection. Researchers are still looking for various cancer markers in the blood released from the cancer. Some of the commonly practiced tests are the cancer antigen 125 (CA 125) test for ovarian cancer, cancer antigen 15-3, cancer antigen 27-29 for breast cancer, cancer antigen 19-9 for pancreatic cancer, alpha-fetoprotein (AFP) for liver cancer, calcitonin for thyroid cancer, human chorionic gonadotropin (HCG), Prostate-specific antigen (PSA).

Liver function test

The liver function tests tell us how well the liver is functioning. This test looks for the protein and enzyme levels produced or cleared by the liver. Some of these proteins are alanine aminotransferase (ALT), aspartate aminotransferase (AST), alkaline phosphatase (ALP), and gamma-glutamyl transferase (Gamma GT). You don't have to remember these big terms; they are proteins released from the liver. Due to some blockage (caused by a tumor or some extra mass) in the liver or the bile duct, they can get stuck in the system, and their levels can get raised.

The liver function test also gives us the level of bilirubin and albumin in the blood. Certain cancers like pancreatic or gallbladder cancers result in abnormalities in bilirubin levels leading to symptoms like jaundice, vomiting, yellowing of the skin, and so on.

Creatinine and kidney function test

Suppose a criminal commits some crime and throws the evidence in a dustbin. The police searched the dustbin, found the evidence, and ultimately caught the criminal. A similar thing happens here. The kidney clears every waste material in our body. Tracking the kidney function may explain what is getting out of our system. Any abnormality in the kidney function can help detect the cancer. The levels of some waste material can go up due to blockage, or the extra waste can be released by cancer.

Blood protein testing

When the police have no evidence against a criminal but from within, they just know who the criminal is. If something is wrong, they start looking for evidence and behaving differently. A similar thing happens to our immune system against certain cancers. For example, our immune system releases specific proteins in the blood in response to certain cancers, including myeloma.

Circulating tumor cells test

Sometimes the blood tests catch the tumor cells red-handed. While traveling or spreading, the cancer cells can be found in the blood sample.

2.7. Cancer scans

Along with the blood tests, the doctor needs to know where the cancer is and how much the tumor has grown before going in for further treatment. Sometimes in blood tests, nothing abnormal is detected during the very early stages of cancer, but the cancer grows. So, the doctor wants some images to see if everything is normal or if any extra mass or lump is present at the suspected place. When we are talking about 'some image of cancer,' we need to understand the limitations of this.

Let's take an example of a crime scene again. Two important limitations of CCTV footage of the crime scene need to be understood. The angle from which the camera is taking the image, also the quality of the image. Even after the footage is there, getting a good-quality image of the criminal is sometimes difficult. Similarly, taking an image inside the body is difficult as light does not pass through our body. That is why we use other forms of energy to get an image of the inside body parts. Doctors recommend different types of scans to get a good-quality tumor image.

Ultrasound scan or USG

In this test, sound takes a picture instead of light. High-energy ultrasound waves are sent inside our body, and they echo off. An image is generated using these echoes of the sound waves. The generated image is called a sonogram.

X-ray scan

In X-ray scans, X Rays (very low radiation) are passed through our body to create an image of the internal organs. During this test, the technician positions the patient's specific organ towards the X-ray beam and then runs the scan. The patient must be still during the process and might have to hold their breath for some time. Even though the X-ray uses very low radiation, it is not considered harmful.

Bone scan

Bone scans are specific tests for bone cancers. They are useful for detecting bone cancers and any bone damage or abnormality.

CT scan

A CT or computed tomography scan is a series of X-ray scans from different angles. This technology uses an X-Ray machine connected to a computer that takes images of the same organ from different angles. Then it uses all these images to understand the area better in three dimensions (3D). The machine looks like a doughnut, and the patient lies inside while the machine moves around the patient's body.

MRI scan

MRI, or magnetic resonance imaging, uses magnets to take images of the internal organs. In this scan, a high-powered magnet and radio waves are used to take images as slices of the whole organ, and then these images are used to form a 3D image of the organ. The MRI scans are usually very clear, and the shape and size of the tumor are spotted easily.

Nuclear scan

A radioactive material is used for this specific scan. Before the scan, a small amount is injected into the patient. This material then travels through the blood to get collected at specific organs. The radiation is recorded afterward to get a picture of the same.

PET scan

Cancer cells use up more glucose than healthy cells. A PET scan or positron emission tomography uses this property of the cancer cells to detect exactly where they reside and where exactly they have spread. In this process, the patient is injected with radioactive glucose that goes to the cancer-specific places and accumulates there. Then the scanner takes images of the cancer cells' locations, giving an exact idea about cancer growth.

2.8. Biopsy

The suspect is innocent until proven guilty. So, even after the blood and imaging tests, a confirmatory test is called a biopsy. This test involves taking samples from the suspected tissue and then studying the cells inside to check if they are cancerous. This test is also called histopathological analysis, as the histology or the internal tissue structure is analyzed. The biopsy is of different types depending on the sample collection process. Some of them are discussed here.

Needle biopsy

This type of biopsy uses a needle-like structure to get tissue samples for analysis. If the needle is very fine, it is called fine needle aspiration biopsy. Sometimes the needle is a little broad to get the deep samples. This type of procedure is called core needle biopsy. Sometimes the tissue that needs to be tested can not be seen from outside. Then the procedure is done with real-time imaging using a CT scan or MRI.

Endoscopic biopsy

An endoscopic biopsy is performed when the sample must be taken from our digestive or respiratory system. In this procedure, a long thin, flexible tube or the endoscope is inserted within our body, and tissue samples from the desired area are collected under continuous medical supervision.

Skin biopsy

The skin biopsy is performed when a tissue sample is taken from the skin. Different types of skin biopsies include shave biopsy, punch biopsy, incisional biopsy, and excisional biopsy. In the shave biopsy, a razor-type instrument is used. For punch biopsy, a small tissue area is cut like a punch. A small part of the tissue is cut using a scalpel for incisional biopsy. The whole lump is removed while performing an excisional biopsy.

Bone marrow biopsy

Bone marrow biopsy is recommended for blood cancers when the cancer cells are present within the bone marrow. A long needle is inserted inside the suspected bone, and the sample is taken for further analysis.

Surgical biopsy

When surgery is done to get the sample for biopsy, when any other way is not possible to check the cancer, this procedure is considered.

2.9. AI-based cancer detection

Artificial intelligence (AI) is a hotcake problem solver and has been widely popularized in recent years. These are algorithms where an enormous amount of data from cancer patients is used to create these programs which can detect the possibility of developing cancer. These AI-based techniques mostly rely upon image-based tests. Mammograms are already used for breast cancer scans to understand the risk of getting cancer. Pap scans do the same for cervical cancers. These techniques help diagnose several cancers even before the disease has appeared.

Robust research is going on to use these techniques in cancer detection. They can prove to be of great help to doctors with lesser experience and will be able to save a lot of time and money. Sometimes in lung cancer, some scans look like cancerous growths when they are not. These false results can also be reduced by using AI-based tools. But some restrictions are coming into focus nowadays. These AI-based techniques are so new that they are still not practiced on a large scale. Also, these AI-based results depend on the programming and the data used to design them. For example, suppose some AI-based techniques are developed using the reports of white people. In that case, they will not necessarily show accurate results for black or Asian people. Of course, these AI-based techniques or their developers are not being racist here. But the lack of data availability and genetic differences play a crucial role. But all these limitations can be taken care of, and according to doctors, in the future, AI will help us to detect cancer in much easier ways.

2.10. When should you consult a doctor

We must be aware of our bodies to detect cancer early and easily. We are the best people who know our bodies very well. We should not ignore any persistent change that happens. Maybe that small change can detect cancer early when a cure is easy and possible. In the next chapter, we will discuss some cures for cancer.

* * *

SECRET NO. 2: BREAKING THE MYTHS

"Healing Happily! Let's cure cancer together" Ayaan looked at the poster with a patient smiling at him as if the doctor in front had cracked a joke. These cancer hospitals make their posters as if one is lucky to have cancer. Since Ayaan got the news, he can not sleep or think of anything else. What to tell his father? How is Maa going to react? Her hypertension problem should not be affected again.

Naina and Ayaan's sister Mausam came to him. "We saw the hospital facilities. The arrangements are nice," said Naina. "We should talk to the doctor to start without further delay," Mausam said. Ayaan nodded, still gazing at the poster before them, hoping his father would get the best treatment there.

* * *

3. Cure for Cancer: The Sorcerer's Stone

Cancer is not only a disease. It is a group of many diseases. Do we expect one single medicine to cure hundreds of diseases? Then why is the expectation so different for cancer? Cancer varies from patient to patient and tumour to tumour. Other factors affecting cancer include immunity, age, stress level, etc. Every other day in a different newspaper article, we read that scientists have found some substances that have anti-cancer properties and expect a miraculous cure for cancer. When that does not happen, we lose hope and start fearing cancer even more. The rationale of this chapter is to clear some frequently misunderstood facts about cancer.

3.1. Is there any actual "Cure" for cancer?

People fear cancer because everyone knows there is no "cure" for cancer. Still, everyone wants the doctor to say this magical word. And the doctor never says it. Yes, cancer does not have any cure as of now. But that does not mean anyone who gets cancer will never be cured from cancer. Cancer treatments depend heavily on the type of cancer and the patient's condition. So, one should not fear cancer because there is no magic potion to heal all types of cancer for all patients. Instead, one should start the treatment immediately to ensure the best cure.

3.2. Why is it so hard to cure cancer?

The problem of cancer treatment is the diversity of the cancers. There are hundreds of diseases within cancer; the cancer cells are also our cells. So the treatment must be very specific for the cancer cells, leaving the normal cells behind. Such specific medicine development is very difficult. Different cancer cells also respond differently depending on the patient's condition. Besides, cancer cells are very robust while growing. They can survive in very harsh conditions, making it even more difficult to kill them.

3.3. Can cancer be cured without medication?

Conventional drugs or medications used in cancer treatments are mostly chemicals that cause harmful side effects. Some alternative medications have helped to improve patients' conditions. These alternate medications include yoga, and mind-body therapies, to name a few. There needs to be more research and proof that they work. But these are not enough to treat cancer without other therapies. These alternate medicines can help in the recovery process. One should always consult a qualified medical doctor before making any such decision.

3.4. Is there a 100% cure for cancer?

Cancer can be 100% cured for individual patients. It depends on the patient's condition, the stage at which the cancer was detected, and the type of cancer. But this does not mean all cancers for all patients are 100% curable. As the treatment is difficult for cancer, 100% cured patients are less. A 100% cure is possible, and many patients have been cured of cancer completely. But cancer is a condition where some cells remain that can grow back and form tumours. So there is a chance of getting the cancer back.

3.5. How long do cancer survivors live?

Cancer survivors are the people who have had cancer, and after treatment, no signs of cancer are present in their bodies. One can also consider people living with cancer under regular checkups as cancer survivors. Survival after cancer depends on the patient's health conditions, how well the cancer treatment has happened, and the type of cancer. The number of survivors after cancer has grown recently due to the current use of advanced therapies. The patient's survival rate also depends on the patient's age. Doctors generally suggest the patient would live 5 years and more after successful cancer treatment for aged people. But there are cases when people survive for more than 20 years after cancer treatment.

3.6. What are some most curable cancers?

The cure for cancer depends upon the patient's health, the stage at which it is detected, and the type of cancer. Still, some cancers have better success rates than other types of cancers to cure. Some of them are breast cancer, prostate cancer, uterus cancer, testicular cancer, thyroid cancer, melanoma, cervical cancer, and Hodgkin's lymphoma when they are diagnosed at stage 1 or stage 2. Cancer screenings are proving to be very useful in treating these cancers. Other cancers are also curable depending on how much the tumour has spread.

3.7. Does cannabis work on cancer?

Some people claim that cannabis is helpful in cancer treatments, and people who use it have gotten good results by using it. Though there is no scientific proof that it helps treat cancer. Bearing the pain of cancer treatment does get easier after using cannabis. So, some doctors may suggest it with other pain relievers when no other options are left. The side effects of cancers can be helped by cannabis or different products from cannabis.

3.8. Can Ayurveda or homoeopathy cure cancer?

Ayurveda and homoeopathy do not cure cancer. Some of the practitioners claim that they can cure cancer. Still, they are mostly similar to the alternative treatments given to the patients if no other treatment options are available. These therapies' substances might have anticancer effects, but the mechanism is still unknown. So, even if someone claims to get results, the confidence level of that result needs to meet statistical significance levels. Studies have shown that regular practitioners of Ayurveda and homoeopathy must be more confident about the exact mechanism of action and risk factors associated with their therapies. Most ayurveda and homoeopathy practitioners (97% and 84%) want to know more about cancer. So, taking these two therapies to cure cancer should be done carefully, considering all the risks.

3.9. Is there a natural remedy?

Just because something is natural does not mean it is good for our health. Sometimes natural products can also interact with our normal physiology and cause problems. So any natural remedies one might think of practising should be consulted with the doctor first. Many natural products have been shown to have anti-cancer properties. They can be helpful along with the treatment provided by health professionals. The main problem with these natural products is that research is still going on for their anticancer effects. So, how exactly they work and possible side effects are still under research.

3.10. How close is medical science to finding a cure for cancer?

Despite spending thousands of dollars on cancer research, we still do not have that medicine with Mida's touch that can cure cancer overnight. But significant advancement has been made in this field. The rate of patients' survival has increased a lot in the previous years. Treatment of different cancers has also progressed, especially with targeted therapy, immunotherapy, etc. In the next chapter, different types of cancer treatments are discussed. To answer the question, we can say that the journey is yet to be finished, but we have come far from where it started.

* * *

SECRET NO.3: DOWN THE RABBIT HOLE (TREATMENT)

"Well then, let's start the treatment, Mr. Ayaan. From the scans, we can see all the tumours. We will operate them and send them for a quick biopsy. This way, we can understand how much the cancer has spread. If it is treatable, we will continue the surgery. If we see that the situation is out of our hands, we will have to stop the surgery in between and think of other treatments," said the doctor.

Ayaan was startled by the idea of the doctor cutting open his father and doing all this. He knew there was no other way, and he nodded, having complete faith in the doctor." When are you planning for the operation?" he asked. The doctor told his secretary to get everything done, and he will do the surgery as early as possible. Ayaan helplessly asked, "Will he be fine after the operation?" The doctor said he would try his best.

Ayaan came back to the hospital bed where Mr Rao was staying. He was cracking jokes and laughing with Naina and Mausam. Ayaan looked at them and smiled. He just wanted to freeze this moment forever as he didn't know what the future held.

* * *

4. Therapies and medications for cancer

Once the patient gets diagnosed with cancer, most doctors suggest treatment as soon as possible. The cancer will not rest but keep spreading. The treatment depends on the patient's age, health condition, and cancer stage. The commonly used treatments are discussed in this chapter.

4.1. Why are cancer therapies, not cures?

When we talk about cancer treatments, they are essentially different from cancer cures. These treatments or therapies can cure individual patients' cancer. Still, these therapies are not the ultimate cure for cancer. The therapies against cancer are different for each patient and their cancer stage. So the doctors decide the best therapies for individual patients during the treatment. Some common therapies are discussed in detail below.

4.2. Chemotherapy

Whenever we think of cancer treatments, our brain automatically connects it to the word "chemotherapy". It has been practiced for a long time. Let's understand how chemotherapy works. You must have noticed many cancer survivors becoming bald after getting cancer. That level of hair loss happens due to chemotherapy and not because of cancer itself. In chemotherapy, doctors prescribe some drugs which are made of harmful chemicals. Because these are chemicals, the name of this treatment is chemotherapy. Chemicals do not distinguish between normal and cancer cells, so they kill everything. Imagine blasting a small bomb to eliminate mosquitoes at home. You will eliminate the mosquitoes, but other things will also get damaged. Chemotherapy causes something similar to the human body. The doctors decide on chemotherapy dosages for individual patients depending on how much they need and can take. There are a lot of side effects of chemotherapy, making the treatment even more miserable than cancer.

4.3. Radiotherapy

In radiotherapy, our body is exposed to harmful radiation that changes our genes. This change ultimately kills cancer cells. The radiation does not kill the cancer cells immediately; it can also kill them after a few weeks and months after treatment. Imagine having a radioactive substance with you that will kill the cancer cells and affect the healthy cells. This type of treatment involves radiation, which also causes harmful side effects.

4.4. Surgery

When a patient is lucky, they can avail the option for surgery. The doctor recommends surgery depending on the patient's health and cancer stage. The doctor removes the cancerous tissue from the patient's body during this process. Sometimes patients undergo severe deterioration after surgery, depending on their health conditions. Most of the time, if the surgery is successful, the patient recovers from cancer. But the risk of getting cancer back after surgery is there as it is not easy to eradicate all the cancerous cells from the body. If some cancerous cells remain inside, they can still grow, and cancer can return. To minimize the risk of cancer recurrence, doctors often recommend chemotherapy sessions to kill those undetected possible cancer cells.

4.5. Hormone therapy

Some cancers use hormones to grow and spread. For these cancers, doctors use hormone therapy. They stop the production of those hormones that are being used up by cancer. This way, our body cuts off water and food to the enemies or the cancer to stop its growth. But as they involve normal hormone production of our system, it causes side effects. Side effects are different for every cancer type and may vary in males and females.

4.6. Immunotherapy

Our immune system is present to defend us against all abnormal types of cells. The cancer cells are smart enough to bypass the immune system and have their ways. In immunotherapy, the doctors provide our immune system with that "extra help" to identify the cancer cells. This therapy activates our immune cells against the cancer cells. Immunotherapy is a highly emerging field that is being used in modern treatments. It has very less side effects than other conventional methods.

4.7. Stem cell transplant

Stem cells are the mother of different cell types. They are like children who can become whatever they want when growing up. Stem cells are special cells that can grow into any cells they want, including blood, skin, lung, etc. A stem cell transplant is not used to treat cancer directly. They are used for the recovery of the cells after treatment. As a side effect of chemotherapy, all the stem cells in the body might die. This results in no new cell formation. The stem cell transplant is used then.

4.8. Targeted therapies

Cancer cells use certain specific proteins to grow and communicate with each other. Targeted cancer therapy disrupts this communication and growth by disturbing these cancer-specific proteins. The targeted therapies vary depending on the type of cancer. Many researchers are still going on to understand how these proteins work and how they can be used against cancer growth.

4.9. Combination therapy

The cancer treatments that are practiced by doctors nowadays are mostly a combination of different therapies that are present. They decide the best possible treatment depending on the patient and cancer stage. For example, after surgery, doctors often suggest chemotherapy to ensure the damage of all the cancer cells in the body.

4.10. Other therapies in use

Other than these types of treatments, doctors also recommend other therapies, including gene therapy, hyperthermia and photodynamic therapy. Gene therapy is used to change the genes to treat cancer. The genes responsible for cell death are introduced in the cancer cells, and that's how they start to die. In the case of hyperthermia, the cancerous tissue is heated to 113°F to kill cancer cells inside the body. Photodynamic therapy uses a drug which radiates light and goes to kill the cancer cells specifically.

To summarize, modern treatments used for cancer are emerging daily. New researches continue to improve the therapies and their success rates. Hopefully, the cure rates will increase very shortly.

* * *

SECRET NO. 4: RAY OF HOPE
(RIGHT GUIDANCE)

"Should we go for a second opinion?" Ayaan asked at the dinner table. They were eating at the hospital canteen. "We cannot just blindly trust this one doctor before he operates Father," he added. Now that the jaundice is in control, he looks fine from the outside. He had also known some cases where the patients could not survive significant surgery. He remembered how Aunt Lata died because of the treatment and not directly because of the cancer. They believe she would have survived more if they did not let the doctor operate on her. But now, what should he do?

Naina was also thinking of getting a second opinion before the operation. She had already sent the reports to a doctor friend. He also suggested an operation. But still, another doctor should confirm before the operation. Mausam knows many doctors there. She took an appointment with another doctor.

They met the second doctor the next day, who confirmed an operation was needed. He recommended the first doctor for the operation. He also suggested the hospital where the best facility at the best price would be available. Finally, they decided on a date for the operation and to face fate together, whatever and however it was.

* * *

5. Importance of the proper guidance

Proper guidance is crucial in cancer treatment. Cancer is a complex and challenging disease that requires accurate information, expert advice, and appropriate guidance throughout its diagnosis, treatment, and survivorship phases. Decisions need to be made in so many different ways. Where the treatment will be performed, financial issues, which option is best for the patient, and which doctors to consult. The following are some key reasons why proper guidance is crucial in cancer treatment.

5.1. Cancer Awareness

Cancer information can be confusing and overwhelming. The proper guidance can help individuals and their families understand their type of cancer, treatment options, potential side effects, and long-term prognosis. By doing so, they can make informed decisions about their treatment and better understand their disease.

5.2. Having a clear idea about the condition

Cancer patients can access the right resources and support services with the proper guidance. Help may include:
- Navigating the healthcare system.
- Obtaining financial support for treatment.
- Obtaining palliative care.
- Finding support groups.

Cancer patients benefit from such guidance since it optimizes their overall care experience.

5.3. First thing to do after cancer detection

Expert medical advice should be sought immediately after cancer detection. Consult an oncologist or cancer specialist to discuss your diagnosis, treatment options, and next steps. You will receive valuable information and guidance tailored to your situation. Ensure you receive the best possible care by consulting with healthcare professionals specializing in your type of cancer. Participate in your treatment decision-making by asking questions, seeking a second opinion, and actively participating. The fight against cancer depends on early intervention and comprehensive healthcare.

5.4. Few terms you must know about

Understanding cancer terms can assist individuals in navigating conversations with healthcare providers, comprehending medical information, and actively participating in their care. Here are a few cancer terms explained:

Tumor: An abnormal mass of cells that may be cancerous (malignant) or non-cancerous (benign). Invading tissues and spreading to other parts of the body are cancer risks.

Metastasis: When cancer spreads to other organs. Cancer cells can spread through the bloodstream or lymphatic system, forming new tumors.

Carcinoma: A cancer that begins in the epithelial cells, which line the body's internal and external surfaces. Most cancers, including breast, lung, and prostate, are carcinomas.

Sarcoma: Cancer of connective tissues, like bones, muscles, and fat. Sarcomas are less common than carcinomas but can occur anywhere.

Biopsy: Examining tissue or cells under a microscope to determine if there is cancer or other abnormality.

Chemotherapy: The process of using powerful drugs to kill or halt the growth of cancer cells in the body. It is often combined with other cancer treatments and can be administered orally, intravenously, or topically.

Radiation Therapy: Shrinking or destroying tumors with high-energy radiation, such as X-rays. The treatment is typically targeted at the cancerous area.

Remission: A state in which no signs or symptoms of cancer are present. Remissions can last for a short time (partial remission) or a long time (complete remission), but they do not guarantee a cure.

Palliative Care: Care provided to individuals with serious illnesses, including cancer, to improve their quality of life. The treatment aims to manage symptoms, relieve pain, and address emotional and social concerns.

Survivorship: This phase of cancer care begins after treatment and continues throughout a person's life. During follow-up, recurrences are monitored, late effects of treatment are managed, and overall well-being is promoted.

A few examples of cancer terms you may hear are listed here. For a complete understanding of specific terms associated with an individual's diagnosis and treatment, it's crucial to consult healthcare professionals and reputable sources.

5.5. Is the treatment more dangerous than the cancer itself?

When a child refuses to take medicines, does he think his disease is better than the medicine? The situation is somewhat similar here. As the medicine tastes bitter, the child might not like it. But to get well soon, it is essential. Similarly, cancer treatment is painful many times, especially during chemotherapy. The side effects of the chemicals cause the pain. Scientists are trying to minimize the side effects as much as possible, but severe side effects can still be observed. Cancer cells are killed during chemotherapy using small doses of dangerous chemicals. These chemicals do not distinguish between healthy and cancer cells leading to the death of critical healthy cells. Some side effects include extreme pain, nausea, sore throat, infertility, fatigue, constipation, diarrhea, etc. But most of the cancer treatment plans also cover the recovery of the side effects of cancer therapies.

In most cases, separate sets of specialized persons are available who handle the side effects of the existing treatment plan. Just like that kid who doesn't want to get cured of his disease because the medicine tastes bitter, many patients might fear the side effects of the cancer treatment. But it is always wise to go for the treatment as survivorship can improve significantly if the patient undergoes cancer treatment.

5.6. Finance matters

While talking about the severity of cancer, the cost of the treatment is also a part of the nightmare. Knowing the treatment cost is very important regardless of whether one is financially healthy or worried about money. Cancer treatment is costly, and worrying about the cost is very natural. Here are some ways to manage the treatment cost.

- Health insurance is vital in cancer treatments. Insurance companies usually cover a part or the entire treatment cost depending on the insurance policy.
- Before starting the treatment, a total estimated cost should be asked from the hospital.
- Talking to the doctor helps a lot. Sometimes if the doctor knows about the patient's financial problems, the treatment plan is chosen accordingly. It does not mean that treatment quality will be compromised.

- Always cross-checking the hospital bills is necessary. This way, a clear understanding of the expense can be achieved.
- Search for available patient groups and organizations that help cancer patients financially. Sometimes the patient's employer or family member also helps with the treatment costs.

5.7. Informed Decision

Making decisions can sometimes be very difficult for cancer patients and their families. Anxiety, unfamiliar medical terms, probability, and urgency complicate this decision-making. All the decisions should be made in a calm and aware mindset. Here are a few things one needs to remember before making a decision.

- The patients and their close ones should know their health condition and cancer stage. This understanding helps when making a decision.
- The risk factors associated with the treatment should be discussed in detail with the doctors. The quality of life before and after treatment should be taken into account.
- Understanding priorities at that moment makes the decision-making process much more manageable. It helps the patients to be practical while making a decision.
- Financial conditions and the chances of a better life after treatment must be consulted with the doctors before decision-making.

- Discussing the condition with a wise and trustworthy person (preferably outside the family who may be a good friend) can help decision-making. They can give input without being emotional while making the decision.

5.8. Identifying the proper guidance

The proper guidance can help the patient and significantly change the treatment outcome. Most importantly, the patient should consult a good doctor who is wise and knowledgeable about current therapies and technologies. After identifying the source of the cancer, the patient should consult an experienced doctor practicing on that specific organ. Apart from that, one can also consult a group of specialists in radiology, chemotherapy, and surgeons who can provide a comprehensive perspective on the treatment plan. Tapping into reliable sources of information such as journals and books can increase knowledge and help make an informed decision.

5.9. Do you need a second opinion

Anyone can make mistakes, even doctors. It is always good to have a second or third opinion. Doctors can guide patients based on their experience and skills, which can vary from doctor to doctor. Taking a second opinion allows the patients to understand the condition better. They can have better peace of mind to make an informed decision about the treatment plan. It helps to reduce the chance of misdiagnosis, and patients are empowered to participate actively in the treatment process.

5.10. How much time should you invest

'The clock is always ticking'. A lot of anxiety grasps the patients because of the feeling of urgency while making decisions. Taking a second or third opinion is an excellent option, and understanding the situation is also a crucial step in the treatment. However, one should save time while gathering knowledge and information. The decision must be made depending on the cancer stage and health condition. This time may vary for individual patients. Consulting the doctors and making informed decisions must be done as soon as possible.

Proper guidance is essential in cancer care by providing accurate information. It also helps by supporting treatment decisions, addressing emotional needs, connecting individuals with resources, and facilitating survivorship. With confidence and support, patients can actively participate in their care, make informed decisions, and navigate the cancer journey.

* * *

SECRET NO. 5: KEEP CALM AND FIGHT CANCER

*I*t was a day before the operation. All the loved ones of Mr. Rao came to spend some good times with him. The whole family was there with him. Mr. Rao was tensed, but he was not showing it. He was trying to crack jokes like he used to do throughout his life, but no one found them funny that day. Mr. Rao was repeatedly asking Ayaan about the exact details of the operation. He was coming up with new doubts each time about what the doctor had already discussed with them. Everyone was serious that night. Ayush, the 5-year-old son of Mausam, was also quiet that day. Somehow he also knew that something about the day was not okay, and everything felt so gloomy.

Mrs. Rao hugged her husband privately before they left for the hospital the next day. She told her husband, "Fight dear, fight and win this war. Remember how I used to wait for you every night when you came home after a long day at the office. Some days, you were late. But you have always come back. After this war is over, YOU come home to ME. I'll be waiting". A drop of tear rolled down Mr. Rao's chin. He kissed goodbye to his wife and left for the battle that he had ahead.

* * *

6. Mindset of cancer

Mindset is the way of looking into something. It is a belief that a person has about the way natural processes work. Looking at things from a different perspective can result in totally different outcomes. Cancer patients often see cancer as associated with all the negativities, ultimately leading to anxiety and depression. Half of the cancer battle is won if one can overcome this harmful mindset related to cancer.

6.1. Don't panic

The detection of cancer is overwhelming news not only for the patient but for their loved ones as well. In such situations, most people face extreme responses like panic attacks. Panic attacks bring extreme emotions of anxiety and trauma at a time that causes the patients to feel overwhelmed. Some common symptoms of a panic attack are dizziness, shortness of breath, pounding heart rates, trembling, sweating, chest pain, and so on. Overcoming the panic situation is very important for the patient's overall health.

Imagine a family with a lot of differences. Everyone is fighting with each other. If someone wants to attack that family and fraud them, it will be effortless for the criminal to do so. Because, unlike a happy and healthy family, here people are fighting with each other, and they are not united or trust each other. The same thing happens to a cancer patient who is panicking. That way, the patient ends up helping the cancer to grow.

6.2. Importance of positive thinking

In a battle, if someone starts to think that they are weaker than the enemy, they will lose the battle. Their thoughts will be responsible for the consequences. Instead, if someone focuses on their strong points, they will at least have the courage to fight. Similarly, if someone thinks about the negative impacts of cancer, they might lose the battle before even fighting it. Focusing on somewhat better things provides courage and the chances of recovery increase.

6.3. Can a positive mindset cure cancer

Curing cancer just by having positive thinking is not evidenced scientifically. However, it helps in the recovery of cancer patients. Patients with a positive mindset recover better as they don't have to face internal trouble and anxiety.

6.4. How to remain positive after cancer detection?

It is easier to say than to do. Having a positive mindset can sound more theoretical than actually practicable. However, being positive does not mean being happy and cheerful about cancer; being positive means accepting the situation. At the moment of cancer detection, one need not think about all the negative things that might happen in the future. One can also focus on the positive changes that might occur in their life. There are a few things one might practice to remain positive.

- Having a journal might help.

- Focus on the things you can control and be more hopeful.
- Don't overthink and think about the present situation instead of the future.
- Find people who are always there for you and spend quality time with them.

6.5. Positive people around you

Having positive people around you might help in cancer treatment. It does not control the tumor or the therapy, but the patient can feel better and comfortable surrounded by people they love. This way, the patient's mind can divert from cancer, and its negative impacts, and also, being in a positive environment can help them focus on the positive aspect of life. The hope they might get from the people surrounding them might help them achieve a positive attitude by keeping them away from anxiety and panic attacks.

6.6. How does laughter help?

It is proven that laughter helps to produce positive changes in human emotions. After a good laugh, people feel lighter and, most importantly, better. In cancer treatment, many hospitals use laughter as a therapy named humor therapy as a treatment to keep patients happy. Laughter therapy is also used to help patients to cope with extreme pain caused by cancer treatment. This therapy mainly uses jokes, funny movies, and hilarious stories. The vital aspect of laughter therapy is that our body can not differentiate between a real and a fake laugh. The body produces the same substances as a response to the movement of facial muscles and the sound of laughter. So even if the joke is not good, one might want to fake a laugh for the therapy to work.

6.7. Can cancer be a good thing?

Human life is unpredictable anyway; why should one worry about cancer? Worrying will help the cancer grow even faster. Cancer is what it is. But it is up to us how we take it. Cancer comes with a negative mindset, and people see it as the worst catastrophe of their life. Cancer is not a good thing, but one might take it as an opportunity to look at life from a different perspective which wasn't possible otherwise. No one can change the future. But our mindset today decides the fate of tomorrow. Facing cancer with a positive outlook can help the patient to survive better, and the chance of a cure is increased with a positive attitude.

6.8. Why does cancer change life?

Cancer is overwhelming for the patient as well as for their loved ones. While cancer affects a person physically and mentally also, many changes happen. While coping with cancer, many strong feelings can affect the patient, which changes the perspective of life for the patient. Many people feel anxiety and depression while fighting cancer. On the other hand, some people find hope and stick to the good things that might come with cancer. Their point of view in life changes, and most of them start enjoying the little things in life.

6.9. What does cancer teach you?

Surviving cancer teaches different things depending on person to person. But most cancer survivors started to live in the moment after their cancer treatment. Cancer survivors mostly become much more confident about life after their treatment. They become happy in their lives no matter what. When people overcome the fear of death and accept life with all difficulties, they start appreciating the beauty of the little things. Cancer survivors are real heroes, and their way of looking at life is something everyone should assimilate into.

6.10. Is there any scientific proof of a positive mindset beating cancer

Having a positive attitude does not directly have any effect on cancer. Nobody got a complete cure by having just a positive attitude. However, it helps the cancer journey to be more accessible. The hope of becoming better and defeating cancer gives the patients a burning courage that helps them fight cancer. Their mind and body respond in such a way that the therapy becomes effective practically. At least having a positive perspective does not harm the patient, which negative thinking does.

* * *

SECRET NO. 6: STRESS, STRESS, GO AWAY!

*"**P**atient no. 32!" shouted the nurse in the waiting area where Ayaan and family were sitting along with the relatives of other patients. The Doctor was inside the operation theatre, and he had mentioned that the operation would take around 8-10 hours. Everyone from the family was hoping that the Doctor would complete the operation. The Doctor would only understand Mr Rao's stage after opening the area.*

A woman sitting beside Naina ran to the nurse. She is the wife of patient no. 32. After 5 minutes, she returned to the waiting area, crying. Mausam wanted to comfort her and came closer. She was embarrassed by the fact that she was crying in public. But she couldn't help it., her husband returned to his senses after three days. She hugged Mausam, a total stranger, and let it all out. The whole family could feel her pain and happiness at that moment. While listening to her story, Mausam wished her father, too, would return to his senses soon. Was it only Mausam? Everyone in that waiting room thought the same about their loved ones.

* * *

7. Stress! The Best Friend of cancer

Stress is the worst enemy of humankind. Because of the recent hectic lifestyle, stress has become an integral part of our daily life. Essentially stress is how our body responds under pressure. Stress is prevalent in cancer patients because of the overwhelming cancer detection and treatment process. Stress becomes a constant companion not only to cancer patients but to caregivers too. Let's understand stress in detail to avoid it as much as possible.

7.1. What is stress

Stress is a condition of worrying or being under pressure. Stress does affect our physical and mental health. A little stress is good for our day-to-day activities, but much stress is not good. Some symptoms of stress are anxiety, nervousness, inability to relax, stomach upset, body pain, and so on. When our body feels under pressure, it secretes stress hormones such as norepinephrine and epinephrine. These hormones affect our system by causing changes such as an increase in heart rate, blood pressure, and blood sugar levels which ultimately cause problems.

7.2. Stress vs. anxiety

Anxiety is a response that occurs because of stress. The two terms are similar to each other, but there is a fine line between the two. Stress can occur temporarily because of some work pressure, deadline, etc., or in long-term or chronic situations due to chronic illness. While stressed, people face many physiological symptoms similar to anxiety symptoms. Unlike stress, anxiety is a reaction when one always feels anxious, even without a valid stressor present. Overcoming both is crucial, especially in cancer, as they help it grow faster.

7.3. Does stress help cancer

Studies suggest that stressful conditions can help cancer cells spread faster. There are studies where mice with tumours have been kept under stress along with mice without stress, and it was found that mice with stress grew the tumour faster than the control sets. Also, statistics suggest people with stressed conditions develop faster cancer growth.

7.4. Science behind stress helping cancer

During stressful conditions, our body releases some stress hormones, such as epinephrine and norepinephrine. These hormones help in cancer cells' growth. They help the cancer cells to multiply more, and they also help in new blood vessel formation in the tumour so that the cancer cells get ample nutrition. They also activate neutrophils, a type of immune cell that might help the cancer cells grow. Sometimes they awaken the dormant cancer cells by helping them grow faster. Sometimes stress releases steroid hormones that stop cancer cell death and thus help cancer.

7.5. Can only stress cause cancer

There is no such study that proves that taking stress causes cancer. It is not true that if one undergoes chronic stress, it will lead to cancer. But, taking stress may result in our choices of lifestyle which might help in cancer formation. For example, suppose a person is stressed and starts smoking or drinking alcohol regularly. In that case, their chances of developing cancer can increase.

7.6. How to manage stress in cancer

Stress management is an essential aspect while fighting cancer. Stress helps cancer, so the patient not only has to fight cancer, they have to fight stress too. Social and emotional support is critical while managing stress during cancer. Studies suggest that social support lowers the stress hormone level that helps manage stress. Another crucial factor that helps manage stress is through exercise. Apart from that, one must ask for professional help from a mindfulness coach or professional therapist if necessary.

7.7. Does meditation cure cancer

As stress helps cancer during treatment, it needs to be managed. Meditation is the ice to calm the fire of stress in our bodies. It is proven that meditation reduces stress and anxiety and helps the body to respond to treatment appropriately. Meditation calms the mind down and helps to focus on our well-being. It reduces the level of stress hormones and thus achieves mindfulness.

7.8. Does Yoga cure cancer

Yoga is an ancient form of exercise that helps to calm down the anxious mind. Many cancer patients practice Yoga with other therapies, claiming that Yoga helps them feel relaxed. In the cancer cure process, Yoga does not contribute directly, and there is no such evidence of curing cancer by Yoga only. But generally, it lifts the mood and enhances well-being. Yoga also helps stimulate the nervous system, makes muscles flexible, and relaxes the mind.

7.9. Best exercise for cancer

Any exercise is good for cancer treatment. The important thing is to exercise regularly. Exercise helps to reduce stress and revitalize the body. Exercising during cancer treatment has proven to reduce the days taken for recovery. After cancer surgery or during chemotherapy, the side effects are minimized with the help of exercise. The Doctor suggests exercising as a compulsory therapy for the patients. People with other difficulties, such as heart conditions and diabetes, also can develop cancer. For them exercising has been shown to increase survival. Ultimately, regular walking also can help the patients to recover better. But before starting any exercise, a doctor's consultation is a must.

7.10. How to be consistent in stress management

One day if one suddenly decides to be very obedient and start doing all the possible stress management hacks, it is unlikely that they would stick to their routine. Those routines might become like one of our childhood study resolutions that never became a reality. Being consistent while managing stress can be achieved by absorbing things slowly until they become incorporated into the daily routine.

But still, stress comes and does affect us. But by practising Yoga, meditation, and exercises, one is trained and should feel confident to fight stress.

* * *

SECRET NO. 7: YOU ARE WHAT YOU EAT

*I*t has been 6 hours since the operation started. The Rao family members were taking turns to go for lunch. Ayaan went outside the hospital premises to get some food and fresh air. These few weeks are like a nightmare for him. His boss also calls him daily to ask when he will return to the office. He wonders how the office used to work before he joined. But he is not mentally stable enough to even think about his office now.

He was constantly thinking about the operation and the possible outcomes. What if the operation is not successful? What if the father never returns to normal? Was this decision of surgery correct? He got trapped in the web of negative thoughts that, after some point, his optimistic self reminded him to remain positive and face whatever it was.

Being diverted from those thoughts, he remembered that he needed to meet the insurance department about financial matters and sort things. The bill is increasing in hours, and his insurance limit is also getting over very soon.

While Ayaan was lost in his stressful thoughts, the shopkeeper of the nearby food stall asked him what he wanted to have. Ayaan quickly gazed over the menu loaded with oily and spicy junk foods. He randomly ordered one dish and asked for a cup of tea with a cigarette when the food was being prepared. "My father never smoked nor ate random things like this. What is the point of all that if you get cancer anyway," he thought while lighting his cigarette.

* * *

8. Importance of food in cancer

Food is an important part of our daily life. Whatever we do, we do it for food. Food gives us all the energy that we need. Cancer is an enemy that resides within the patient along with non-cancer cells. When food provides energy to normal cells, cancer cells become mischievous and try to take up all the energy available in the body. This way, they can survive and grow better. It is one of the main reasons for the weakness of most cancer patients. All the energy they are getting is being wasted to nurture the cancer cells. Can certain foods be harmful to cancer patients? How and why? Let's find out in this chapter.

8.1. What is the best food for cancer?

There is no single superfood that can be labelled as the best food for cancer treatment. But citrus fruits help to reduce the risk of cancer. A study from Japan suggested that people who consume citrus fruits 4 to 5 days a week are less likely to develop cancer than those who consume citrus fruits for two or fewer per week. Healthy food can lead to a healthy system and reduce the risk of cancer. Studies suggest that most of the foods that are considered to be 'cancer-fighting foods' are from plant origins and contain phytochemicals. Phytochemicals are plant-origin nutrients that help fight chronic diseases like cancer. A good way to include more such phytochemicals in your diet is to add more colourful vegetables to your plate.

8.2. Can certain food and chemicals cause cancer?

Certain food and dietary products may increase the risk of cancer development. Sometimes we unknowingly consume harmful substances that ultimately can damage our cells and make them cancerous. Some examples of certain foods are fried foods, processed meat, overcooked meat, etc.

8.3. Cigarettes and cancer

We have to start with cigarettes when discussing food and lifestyle causing cancer. Tobacco and its cancer-causing ability are well-advertised, well-known, and worthy of discussion. The smoke from cigarettes contains at least 70 types of harmful chemicals. When someone (the person who is smoking or the person who is around and inhaling the smoke) inhales the smoke, they take up all these chemicals, which travel throughout their body within their bloodstream. These chemicals can cause damage to any cell of the body and can damage the DNA. Most of these chemicals are carcinogens prone to damage the DNA forming cancer.

8.4. Junk food and cancer

Junk foods or oily fried foods are considered to be very unhealthy, and they increase the risk of causing cancer. But what happens when we eat fried foods? What makes them so unhealthy and makes them powerful enough to cause cancer? When any starch is fried, a harmful substance called acrylamide gets produced, which is highly carcinogenic. Acrylamide is such a harmful substance that researchers do not dare to touch it with bare hands when they work with it. Imagine eating this in the form of tasty fries in packed containers. We consume acrylamide and invite cancer within our system while consuming junk foods.

8.5. Do grills and barbecues cause cancer?

When meat is cooked at very high temperatures, especially in flames, two types of carcinogens are known to be produced: Polycyclic aromatic hydrocarbons (PAHs) and heterocyclic aromatic amines (HCAs). These are two harmful carcinogens that are proven to cause damage to the DNA. So, having meats prepared in direct high flames contain these carcinogens, which increases the risk of cancer development. There is a misconception about microwaves causing cancer due to radiation. But microwaves do not cause radiation outside, and it is not harmful to use them.

8.6. Drinks and cancer

Be it hard or soft, drinks essentially have a role in cancer. Studies suggest that any alcoholic beverage increases the risk of cancer. After alcohol consumption, the human body breaks the alcohol down to form a chemical, acetaldehyde. Acetaldehyde then damages the DNA, which can lead to cancer. Even non-alcoholic drinks, especially packaged cold ones, are unsafe to consume. Most of these cold drinks are coloured with harmful chemicals already proven carcinogens. They also contain preservatives and artificial sweeteners that are even worse for human health.

8.7. How does healthy food fight against cancer?

Where we are blaming some foods for causing cancer, some foods are always fighting for our better health. Such foods include fruits and vegetables. As we have already discussed, phytochemicals help us fight many chronic diseases, including cancer. Another very important substance we get from food is antioxidants. Oxidants are harmful free oxygen that is present within our cells. These oxidants can be generated within us for many reasons, including stress and habits. For example, imagine a small fire within our house. If we don't control the small fire, it can lead to bigger disasters. We can use water or a fire extinguisher to get rid of it. Antioxidants behave like fire extinguishers making the cellular environment calm and peaceful again. Most healthy foods contain these antioxidants, which help to reduce all sorts of oxidant-related problems that might have led to cancer development.

8.8. What to eat to keep cancer away?

It is safe to say that the more natural and colourful your plate is, the lower the risk of developing cancer. Name a few experimentally proven foods that have been shown to lower cancer growth are broccoli, carrots, beans, berries, citrus fruits, tomatoes, garlic, flaxseed, cinnamon, turmeric, nuts, fish containing omega-3 fatty acids and olive oil.

8.9. Plastic in cancer

There is a common use of plastic containers in which food is kept. How safe are those to be used? Let's discuss this in detail. There is no scientific evidence that the plastic containers cause cancer. However, when the food is hot and is stored in these containers, there might be some reaction, and some chemicals from the plastic might get mixed in the food. But the amount of formation of such substances is much less, which is way below the quantity required to cause damage to human beings. Studies suggest that using plastic containers to keep food and drink does not directly cause cancer. On the other hand, the use of plastic is not environmentally friendly and should be cut down.

8.10. Is there a superfood to cure cancer?

Unfortunately, there is no single superfood with healing properties for cancer. However, having vegetables and citrus fruits is helpful in cancer. A balanced diet with more natural and colourful veggies is key to a healthy lifestyle. At the same time, fried starchy foods and overcooked meat should be avoided as much as possible.

* * *

THE SURVIVOR (LIFE AFTER CANCER)

'Ding Dong!' The calling bell of the Rao house rang loudly. Naina and Mrs Rao had been waiting for this moment since this morning. Mrs Rao opened the door and became speechless at what she saw at the door.

The operation was successful, and the doctor released Mr Rao with several restrictions to live life with. He did come back to Mrs Rao after two weeks of his stay at the hospital.

Mrs Rao imagined her husband to be weak after the major operation. Still, the person at the door did not look like her husband. 'What does cancer do to a person!' She wondered, looking at her feeble and trembling husband. Mr Rao was weak, but his eyes showed a stern and proud twinkle. These are the same eyes with the faith and courage that he had while fighting cancer. They have seen worse, but they won the battle. Now it was his time to look back at life with these eyes, wiser than ever.

* * *

9. After treatment care

The post-treatment care is the time when the patience of the patient is being tested. Most of the time, the patient is released from the hospital and needs to be at home with all the post-treatment care required to be provided by the caregivers. A few basic things need to be taken care of after cancer treatment. They are discussed in detail as follows.

9.1. Post-treatment

The cancer treatment process itself makes the patient undergo a series of life lessons. Post-treatment, most patients feel like they are getting a second chance. Cancer teaches them a lot, and after treatment is the time to imply those life lessons. Post-cancer care can be broadly categorized into two groups. First, people who are cancer free and their health condition is like any other non-patient. They must be checked regularly to ensure the cancer is not back. The second type of patients are cancer survivors but with chemotherapy. They need extreme care and protection, and post-cancer care at home becomes very important for these patients and their caregivers.

9.2. Why do patients look devastated after cancer treatment

Imagine the condition of a village after a robust cyclone. Something similar to that happens to the patient during the cancer treatment. The cancer treatment process is exhaustive and extensive. The treatment is severe, and the recovery takes time and, most importantly, patience. Most patients undergo changes in their skin and hair, which they find difficult to accept. But above all, the main thing to remember is that, unlike cancer, they have won the battle.

9.3. Post-treatment symptoms

The post-treatment symptoms may occur depending on what kind of treatment the patient has undergone. Most commonly, patients feel tired and have difficulty in focused thinking. Patients who have undergone surgery may develop symptoms such as infection, scar in the area, nutritional problems, chronic pain, nerve injury etc. Some late effects after chemotherapy include bone and joint pains, muscle weakness, heart problems, kidney disorders, and nerve problems. Radiotherapy also causes post-treatment symptoms like problems with thyroid and adrenal glands, sensitivity, permanent hair loss etc.

9.4. Things to take care of after treatment

Cancer is like that immortal enemy which can come back anytime. Even if someone is declared cancer free, they can again get diagnosed with it. So, one thing to take care of after the cancer treatment is to check once in a while if the cancer is returning. For that, the doctors can advise the best tests to be performed and how frequently one should check. Besides that, overall health should be cared for after cancer treatment. After the cancer treatment, one must do daily physical activity to improve their overall health.

9.5. Importance of Exercise

Exercising is like the sword that one needs to fight cancer. Even when the cancer is not there, one must sharpen the sword daily to be always prepared.

Exercising helps in staying fit and lessens the risk of developing other diseases. The stress and anxiety levels remain under control by exercising daily. Bone and muscle health also develop through daily exercising, which helps in recovery. Breathing exercise also greatly helps during cancer post-treatment care, and the doctors suggest some exercise to strengthen the lungs. It is always very important to consult the doctor about the kind of exercise one should practice.

9.6. Gaining back the health

Cancer treatment changes the patient's overall health, and it is important to regain a healthy lifestyle after cancer treatment. A few things must be taken care of to live a better life even after cancer. Firstly the mental health of the patient needs to be taken care of. The treatment makes the patient emotionally and physically drained, and the survivor needs to become mentally strong and healthy to regain a normal lifestyle. The next important aspect to take care of is the patient's diet. Healthy foods that are carcinogen-free are the best foods for cancer survivors. They are already at risk of getting back cancer, and minimizing the risk is a good approach to live post-cancer treatment.

9.7. Positive thinking

Hope is everything in life. It gives a person the energy and interest to look forward to the future. A person who is a cancer survivor knows how to fight cancer and understands its challenges. But, as the journey is long and tiring, losing hope is common. There will always be some days when negative thoughts approach and make their way through the patients. But the patient needs to overcome the negative thoughts and implement the positive changes that the cancer has taught during its course. Also, no matter how hard it seems, as a cancer survivor, the patient's condition is way better than during the treatment. One needs to remind themselves how far they have come and all the positive things that have happened. This way, the recovery could be faster and less stressful.

9.8. People around you

The mental health of cancer patients depends upon the environment and, most importantly, the people around the survivor. The more positive people are surrounded by the patient giving them more hope and reasons to improve, the better their conditions will be. The recovery speed becomes faster in a positive and healthy, stress-free environment.

9.9. Will cancer come back?

The cancer can technically come back even after years of being cancer free. As the cancer is detected after it is present in a detectable amount, most of the time, very few cancer cells remain in our body which remains undetected. That way, those cells take some time to grow again and form another detectable amount. Sometimes cancer does come back, and sometimes it does not, depending on whether cancer cells are left inside the body even after treatment. That is why doctors suggest screening tests regularly even after cancer is cured.

9.10. Surviving cancer rather than living with it

Even after cancer is cured, the chance of it returning always remains with the patient. So, once a person is diagnosed with cancer, they become used to living with it. At least, the thought of getting back cancer again remains within them always. But "the show must go on, " and life goes on. Accepting the fact makes it easier to handle the cancer.

THE WISH TREE

"Now is the time to understand more, so that we may fear less."

-MARIE CURIE

Ayush was lying on the bed while his grandmother patted his head lightly. She was telling Ayush a fairy tale story. The angel comes and grants three wishes to the princess. Ayush was listening to his grandmother very carefully. His eyes were wide open in excitement to know what would happen next. Who will tell the story's purpose was to let him go to sleep and not away from it? 'What would you have asked from the angel if she granted you one wish?' Mrs Rao asked him affectionately. Ayush said, 'I'll ask the fairy to take cancer away from the world'.

* * *

This chapter is a quick recap on the entire cancer treatment process and dealing with it. It could help to understand how to be aware of one's overall health. It contains a step-by-step plan of action for the cancer treatment approach.

10.1. Early Symptoms

Anything unusual in our changing body can be an early sign of cancer. For example, unusual itching in the skin or the formation of moles growing every day can be a cancer symptom. Weight gain or loss without doing anything can also be an early sign of cancer. We know our bodies best, and the doctor should be consulted if anything unusual is spotted in the body.

10.2. The Detection

The most critical step of cancer treatment is to detect cancer early. After the detection of cancer, the treatment can start. But making sure of the cancer and identifying the exact stage and condition is necessary. One should always be cautious about overall health; if anything seems unusual, one should consult a doctor.

10.3. The Dilemma

Once the cancer is detected, the dilemma and overwhelming feelings of the treatment and huge treatment process a constant fear. But accepting and acting is the right way to deal with the situation.

10.4. The Myths

Cancer detection comes with a lot of advice from people and overwhelming myths about cancer. Understanding the disease and its exact stage is important. One does not need to be a doctor or an expert to have a working understanding of the disease. But knowing the disease and its exact effects could help overcome the fear and ignore the associated myths. This way, one can focus on the truth, not the myths.

10.5. The Decision

After knowing the exact condition of the cancer, the critical step is to decide where the treatment will occur. The patient and their loved ones face many difficulties while making this decision. It is when one needs to calm down and make an informed decision about further treatment. There are many things to decide at this moment. Some important factors to be considered are which doctor to consult, which hospital to proceed with and the finance. The first step should be deciding on a good doctor and consulting the finance matter with the doctor. The doctor might suggest the best possible option for the treatment.

10.6. The Positive People

It is important to stay positive throughout the treatment, which can be achieved by the positive people surrounding the patient. Emotionally and mentally, the whole journey becomes easier if the patient is happy and positive. It decreases stress and helps overcome the situation.

10.7. The Negative People

Human beings are social animals surrounded by positive and negative people. But the more one can avoid negative people, the better it is. People who always make the patient feel bad about their cancer and worry about the future should be avoided as much as possible. This way, the patient's emotional health can deteriorate, impacting the recovery and treatment response.

10.8. The Doctor

The doctor is often considered a lifesaver, and because of the doctors' hard work, millions of people are saved from deadly diseases. So, deciding which doctor to consult is very important in cancer treatment. In cancer treatment, the patient's condition can change within a few minutes, and the doctor needs to decide on instant medications. So, here are a few things that one must look for in their ideal doctor.

- *Experience:* The more experience the doctor has, the better it is. An experienced doctor has faced many patients and can make quick decisions instantly.

- *The specialization* of the doctor also plays an important role. The doctor one is consulting must be an Oncologist or cancer specialist. Even an oncologist can be of different types. So, before deciding which doctor to proceed with for the treatment, ask for the experience record and the doctor's area of specialization.

- *The second opinion* is also very important in cancer treatment, and the doctor consulting for a second opinion should also have good records and experience.

10.9. The Treatment

Once the doctor has decided, the hospital usually takes care of the treatment. During the treatment, one has to follow what the doctors suggest. The caregivers should see that the hospital is correctly attending to the patient and everything is happening with the doctor's advice. Sometimes if the hospital staff cannot attend to the patient all the time because of their other responsibilities and emergencies. Caregivers should always attend to the patient and look for their needs.

10.10. The Post-Treatment

The post-treatment care is the last but not least step of the whole process. It is a time when caregivers play a crucial role for patients. The recovery depends on the post-treatment care, and the patient should feel positive after cancer treatment for a speedy recovery. Friends and family should surround them. They should feel happy and positive this time.

10.11. The Wish Tree

Cancer is a curse to planet Earth and the disease is spreading worldwide. Cancer patients are also increasing daily because of the modern lifestyle and stress. Scientists are trying their best to detect cancer early and to provide necessary treatment. Nowadays, the rate of cancer recovery has increased compared to the past. Constant research is happening to solve cancer-related problems, and doctors are using many newer treatments. It is time that the mentality of cancer being deadly needs to be changed. There are hopes in the field of cancer treatment, and together, we will achieve it. The fight is not easy, but we can not afford to lose the battle against cancer.

84

* * *

ACKNOLEDGEMENT

I bow my head to my family because they showed me the power of unity when the time is worse. I am thankful to the almighty God who gifted me with a wonderful partner as my husband, who is always there by my side. I am a product of all the support given by my parents, parents-in-law, sister, sisters-in-law and brothers-in-law. I am grateful for all the blessings of my five grandparents; I wish you were here to read this book today.

It takes a lot of courage and effort to shape and craft an idea to create a book. I want to thank Inspiring Jatin for his inspiration which made this dream idea take the form of a book.

ABOUT THE AUTHOR

Navodipa B

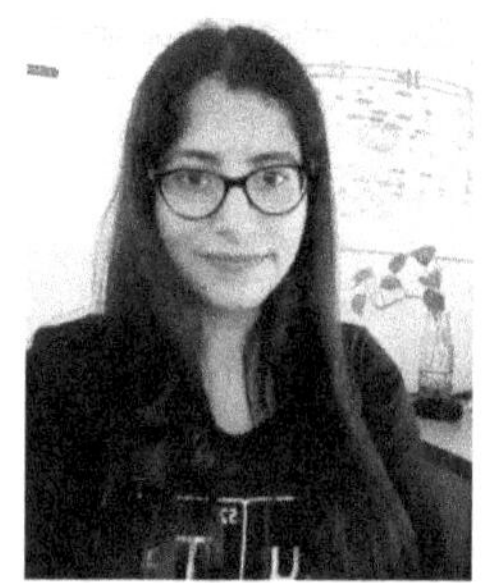

Navodipa B, a passionate advocate, is an expert in biological sciences, driven by a deep desire to combat diseases like cancer. Her doctoral degree in a related field helped her gain a deep understanding of cancer's far-reaching effects. As a cancer patient's caregiver, Navodipa has gained valuable insight into the emotional and physical challenges cancer patients face.

Having encountered cancer patients and their families, Navodipa has dedicated herself to raising awareness about cancer. Her writing aims to empower individuals with knowledge, compassion, and hope, creating a community united against cancer. As a guiding light in the quest for cancer awareness, Navodipa B's work offers hope to those affected by this illness.

www.ingramcontent.com/pod-product-compliance
Lightning Source LLC
Chambersburg PA
CBHW051828250726
48659CB00005B/1737